YELLOW FEVER

TREATING THE ROOT CAUSES OF YELLOW FEVER

DR. AHMED .R

Contents

CHAPTER ONE

INTRODUCTION

The virus that causes yellow fever is carried by a certain kind of mosquito. Both residents and visitors to such regions are affected by the infection, which is most prevalent in parts of Africa and South America.

Yellow fever can produce fever, headache, nausea, and vomiting in moderate cases. However, yellow fever can worsen and result in bleeding (hemorrhaging) as well as issues with the heart, liver, and kidneys. In cases of the most severe variety of yellow fever, up to 50% of patients pass away from the illness.

Yellow fever has no specific therapy. However, you can avoid contracting the illness by having the yellow fever vaccination prior to visiting a region where the virus is known to be present.

Symptoms

You won't exhibit any symptoms or indicators for the first three to six days following the incubation phase of yellow fever. Following this, the infection moves into an acute phase and, occasionally, a potentially fatal toxic phase.

acute stage

Once the illness has progressed to the acute stage, you might notice the following symptoms:

High temperature

Headache

aches in your muscles, especially in your knees and back

Light Sensitivity

vomiting, nausea, or both

appetite decline

lightheadedness

erythematous eyes, lips, or tongue

Usually, these indications and symptoms get better and go away after a few days.

Some patients with acute yellow fever go into a toxic phase after the acute phase, even if symptoms may go away for a day or two. Acute symptoms reappear during the toxic phase, along with increasingly severe and potentially fatal ones. These may consist of:

Jaundice is the yellowing of your skin and the whites of your eyes.

stomach ache and vomiting, occasionally with blood

Reduced need to urinate

Seeing, mouth, and nose bleeding

Bradycardia, or a slow heart rate

Kidney and liver failure

malfunction of the brain, such as delirium, seizures, and coma

Yellow fever's toxic phase can be lethal.

When to visit a physician

Prior to departure

If you are going to a region where yellow fever is known to occur, schedule a visit with your doctor at least four weeks in advance of your trip to discuss whether you should get the vaccine.

Call your physician even if you have fewer than four weeks to get ready. To allow the vaccination to take effect, it is ideal if you can have the shot three to four weeks before to visiting a region where yellow fever is a problem. In addition to offering comprehensive advice on safeguarding your health while traveling overseas, your doctor will assist you in determining whether you require any immunizations.

Following a trip

If you have recently visited an area where yellow fever is known to occur and you start exhibiting symptoms or indicators of the disease's toxic phase, get emergency medical attention.

If you visit to an area where yellow fever is common and you start to exhibit minor symptoms, give your doctor a call.

Aedes aegypti mosquitoes transmit a virus that causes yellow fever. Even the purest water is a breeding ground for these mosquitoes, which multiply in and around human settlements. Tropical South America and sub-Saharan Africa account for the majority of yellow fever cases.

The yellow fever virus primarily infects humans and monkeys. The virus is spread by mosquitoes to humans, monkeys, or both.

The virus spreads through the bloodstream of the mosquito and enters the salivary glands when it bites a human or a monkey carrying the yellow fever virus. The virus enters the bloodstream of the host when an infected mosquito bites a human or another monkey, perhaps leading to disease.

RISK ELEMENTS

If you go somewhere where mosquitoes are still spreading the yellow fever virus, you can get sick. Tropical South America and sub-Saharan Africa are two of these regions.

You may still be at risk even if there aren't any recent reports of infected people in these places. It's probable that local populations are immune to the illness due to vaccinations, or that yellow fever cases haven't been discovered and formally reported.

Obtaining a yellow fever vaccination at least a few weeks prior to your trip can protect you if you intend to visit these regions.

The yellow fever virus can infect anyone, although older people are more likely to become critically ill from it.

COMMITMENTS

Twenty to fifty percent of patients with severe yellow fever die from it. When a yellow fever infection is in its toxic phase, complications can include delirium, coma, kidney and liver failure, and jaundice.

Individuals who survive the infection typically recover over a few weeks to months, often without suffering major organ damage. A person may become fatigued and develop jaundice during this period. Blood infections and pneumonia are examples of secondary bacterial infections that might result in additional difficulties.

Getting Ready for Your Consultation

If you have just returned from a trip overseas and you start experiencing mild symptoms that seem like yellow fever, give your doctor a call. Visit an emergency room, give 911, or dial your local emergency number if your symptoms are severe.

To help you prepare and know what to anticipate from your doctor, here are some details.

Information to obtain beforehand

Symptom history. Jot down any symptoms you've had, together with how long they've persisted.

exposure recently to potential infection sources. Make sure to include all the information about your foreign travels, including the nations you visited, the dates you were there, and any encounters you may have had with mosquitoes.

medical background. List all of your important medical information, including any prescription drugs, vitamins, and supplements you are taking, as well as any other ailments you are being treated for. Your medical professional must also be aware of your immunization history.

queries to put to your physician. To make the most of your time with your doctor, prepare your questions in advance.

You can ask your doctor the following questions regarding yellow fever. Ask as many questions as you like throughout your appointment.

Which of my symptoms is most likely to be the cause?

Are my symptoms coming from any other sources?

Which tests are necessary for me?

Are there any therapies that can aid in my recovery?

How much time do you think it will take to fully recover?

When can I go back to my job or my studies?

Do I run the chance of developing any persistent yellow fever symptoms?

What to anticipate from your physician

You'll probably be asked a lot of questions by your doctor. Being prepared to respond to them could buy you time to go over any topics you'd like to discuss in more detail. Your physician might inquire:

Which symptoms do you have?

When did you start feeling the effects?

Has there been an apparent improvement or worsening of your symptoms?

Did your symptoms go away for a while before returning?

Have you been overseas recently? Where?

During your trip, were you exposed to mosquitoes?

Before your trip, did you get your immunizations updated?

Do you have any additional medical conditions that require treatment?

Do you currently take any medications?

Exams and diagnosis

Yellow fever can be challenging to diagnose based only on signs and symptoms since, in its early stages, it can be mistaken for other viral hemorrhagic fevers, such as dengue fever, typhoid, malaria, and others.

In order to identify your illness, your physician will probably:

Inquire about your past travel and medical experiences.

Get a sample of blood to be tested.

The virus itself may be visible in your blood if you have yellow fever. If not, antibodies and other materials unique to the virus can also be found via blood testing.

CHAPTER TWO

MEDICATIONS AND SUBTLES

There is currently no antiviral drug that effectively treats yellow fever. Because of this, hospital supportive care is the main form of treatment. This include giving oxygen and fluids, keeping blood pressure at a healthy level, replacing lost blood, giving dialysis to patients with kidney failure, and treating any further infections that may arise. Certain individuals have plasma transfusions in order to replenish blood components that enhance coagulation.

In order to prevent spreading the illness to others, your doctor may advise you to stay indoors and away from mosquitoes if you have yellow fever. After contracting yellow fever, you will never again contract the illness.

WAY OF LIFE AND DOMESTIC MEDICINE

Yellow fever is prevented by a highly effective and safe vaccine. Sub-Saharan Africa and certain regions of South America are known to harbor yellow fever cases. See your doctor about whether you require the yellow fever vaccination if you reside in one of these places. Consult your physician at least ten days (ideally three to four weeks) in advance if you intend to travel through these regions. Some nations demand that visitors show a current vaccination record in order to be admitted.

The yellow fever vaccination offers protection for ten years or longer after just one dosage. Typically moderate, side effects can last five to ten days and include headaches, fevers that are low-grade, soreness at the injection site, exhaustion, and muscular stiffness. More serious reactions can happen, usually in children and elderly individuals. These reactions include developing a state resembling true yellow fever, brain inflammation (encephalitis), or even death. The age range for which the vaccination is thought to be safest is nine months to sixty years old.

Consult your physician regarding the suitability of the yellow fever vaccination if you are older than 60 years old, if your kid is under 9 months old, or if you have an impaired immune system.

Defense against mosquitoes

You can help defend yourself against yellow fever by avoiding mosquitoes in addition to receiving the vaccination.

In order to lessen your mosquito exposure:

When mosquitoes are most active, stay indoors and avoid unnecessary activities.

When you enter locations that are infested with mosquitoes, wear long sleeves and long trousers.

Remain in a well-screened or air-conditioned room.

Use bed nets if the air conditioning or window screens in your lodging are inadequate. Pre-treated nets provide an extra layer of security against insects.

Use both of the following while applying repellent to fight off mosquitoes:

Not repulsive to the skin. Put insect repellent with permethrin on your shoes, clothes, camping equipment, and bed netting. Certain clothing and equipment are available for purchase already permethrin-treated. It is not recommended to apply permethrin on human skin.

repellant to the skin. Prolonged skin protection is offered by products containing DEET, IR3535, or picaridin as active components. Based on the number of hours of protection you require, select the concentration. Higher concentrations typically stay longer.

Use only as much chemical repellent as is necessary for the duration of your outdoor experience, keeping in mind that they might be hazardous. DEET should not be applied to small children's hands or to newborns younger than two months. When you're outside, instead, cover your baby's playpen or stroller with mosquito netting.

When used in comparable amounts, oil of lemon eucalyptus, a more natural substance, provides equivalent protection to DEET, according to the Centers for Disease Control and Prevention.

Nevertheless, children under the age of three shouldn't use these goods.

THE END